DECEMBER 2011

NATIONAL INTIMATE PARTNER
AND SEXUAL VIOLENCE SURVEY

Communications Toolkit

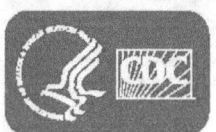

I / Introduction

I. INTRODUCTION

The *National Intimate Partner and Sexual Violence Survey (NISVS)* Communications Toolkit is a practical guide that outlines basic elements for effective communications initiatives: defining a goal or specific objective, identifying your priority audience(s), creating central messages, working with traditional and new media, and mobilizing others. The toolkit contains creative ideas and examples that CDC's partners, grantees, and other groups can use leading up to and following the release of *NISVS* data. Whether you have extensive or little experience with communications, we invite you to use the strategies and materials in this toolkit to promote the *NISVS* data and your organization's commitment to violence prevention.

Sexual violence, stalking, and intimate partner violence are preventable problems. Strategic and sustained communications about why and how these forms of violence occur can change the way people understand and respond to them. Data from *NISVS* will lay the foundation for greater awareness of this long-standing public health crisis and help inform prevention strategies.

● What is the *National Intimate Partner and Sexual Violence Survey*?

The *National Intimate Partner and Sexual Violence Survey* is an ongoing, nationally representative survey that assesses sexual violence (SV), stalking, and intimate partner violence (IPV) among adult women and men in the United States. The primary objectives of the survey are to describe:

- The prevalence and characteristics of sexual violence, stalking, and intimate partner violence
- Who is most likely to experience these forms of violence
- The patterns and impact of the violence experienced by specific perpetrators
- The health consequences of these forms of violence

CDC's National Center for Injury Prevention and Control launched the survey in 2010 with the support of the National Institute of Justice and the Department of Defense. The survey was developed with the help of experts and stakeholders from various organizations and representatives from other federal agencies.

NISVS includes data from English- and Spanish-speaking female and male adults living in the United States and asks respondents about victimization over their lifetime and in the 12 months prior to taking the survey. It captures information on:
- Sexual violence (SV) victimization by any perpetrator, including rape (completed, attempted, and alcohol/drug facilitated forced penetration), being made to penetrate someone else, sexual coercion, unwanted sexual contact, and non-contact unwanted sexual experiences.
- Stalking victimization, including through the use of newer technologies such as text messages, emails, monitoring devices (e.g., cameras and GPS, or global positioning devices), by perpetrators known and unknown to the victim.

- Physical violence by an intimate partner, psychological aggression by an intimate partner, including information on expressive forms of aggression and coercive control, and control of reproductive or sexual health by an intimate partner.

The median length of time to complete the telephone survey in 2010 was approximately 25 minutes. The data represent the national population. Respondents were randomly selected through random-digit dialing of both landline and cell phone numbers.

Financial support from the National Institute of Justice enabled the collection of a separate targeted sample of persons of American Indian and Alaskan Native ethnicity, and the financial support from the Department of Defense enabled the collection of a separate random sample of female active duty military and female spouses of active duty military. Findings from these samples will be described in future publications.

In 2010, a total of 18,049 interviews from the general population sample were conducted. This includes 16,507 completed and 1,542 partially completed interviews. Findings in the 2010 summary report are based on the completed interviews (9, 026 women and 7,421 men).

Why the *National Intimate Partner and Sexual Violence Survey*?

Understanding the magnitude, impact, and consequences of violence against females and males in the U.S. is an important first step in preventing violence. This information can be used to:
- Inform policies and programs that are aimed at preventing these forms of violence
- Provide information for states to consider in their prevention planning and advocacy efforts
- Establish priorities for preventing these forms of violence at the national, state, and local levels

Data collected in future years from the survey can also be used to examine trends in sexual violence, stalking, and intimate partner violence, and to evaluate and track the effectiveness of prevention efforts.

In summary, *National Intimate Partner and Sexual Violence Survey* will help guide and evaluate progress in reducing the substantial health burden from sexual violence, stalking victimization, and intimate partner violence.

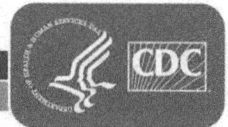

II / Creating a Communications Plan

II. CREATING A COMMUNICATIONS PLAN

Creating a communications plan is essential for achieving the greatest impact from your communications efforts and activities, and it can also support your broader organizational goals and help make the most of resources.

● Steps for Developing a Communications Plan

This step-by-step approach for creating a communications plan may be helpful for responding to the launch of the *National Intimate Partner and Sexual Violence Survey* report and leveraging the data to promote and improve your organization's work to prevent sexual violence, stalking victimization, and intimate partner violence.

Step 1: Define your goal and assess the situation.

NISVS will provide new and compelling information for you to share, but first you must determine what you hope to accomplish in sharing the *NISVS* data. As you set your goal, evaluate the opportunities and challenges your organization faces and the resources available to pursue your goal.

Step 2: Identify your priority audience(s).

Once you've defined your goal, identify the audience(s) you need to reach in order to accomplish your goal. If you identify multiple audiences or segments within each audience, prioritize them, and learn as much as you can about what motivates, influences, and interests them.

Step 3: Develop messages.

After you've identified, prioritized, and gained knowledge about your priority audience(s), develop messages that will resonate with them, compelling them to think, feel, or act in ways that support your goal. Think about the key concepts and language that will resonate with your priority audience(s).

Step 4: Determine strategies and tactics for disseminating your messages.

Determine how your priority audience(s) receive and share information. Think about the best spokesperson, channels, activities, and materials for delivering your messages to your priority audience(s).

Step 5: Create an action plan.

Set your strategies and tactics to a timeline, determining where, when, and how each task will be done. Set milestones and deadlines. Allocate your resources and assign personnel accordingly.

Step 6: Implement, evaluate, and modify your plan.

Before you implement your plan, establish benchmarks and measures by which to evaluate whether or not your plan is meeting your goal and how you will determine success. Once the plan is in motion, if it is not on track to meet your goal, make modifications to your plan to ensure success.

National Center for Injury Prevention and Control

III / Promoting the *National Intimate Partner and Sexual Violence Survey*

III. PROMOTING *NISVS*

NISVS will provide the most current and comprehensive data on SV, IPV and stalking victimization – and an important opportunity to use these data to support your work. Developing a promotional strategy now will position you to lead the conversation about NISVS when it is released and gain exposure for your work on violence prevention.

● Identifying Your Target Audience

Identifying a target audience is a crucial step in any promotion strategy. By establishing which parties will be most interested in, and affected by the NISVS data, you can tailor your campaign to have the largest possible impact.

The key to having a large impact, counter-intuitive as it may seem, is to target a small audience. While you may aspire to have the "general public" talk about your cause, it is next to impossible to find a common denominator for a group so large. A more effective approach is to select a specific audience on whom to focus your communications strategies and to allow the ripple effect to carry your message across waters you alone could not reach.

Follow this step-by-step process to determine your target audience.

Step 1: Name your "Wish List"

If you could convince 500 people to embrace your message today, who would they be? What if you had to narrow down that list to 100 people? What if you had to select only one person to relay your message to? Who would she or he be? Why?

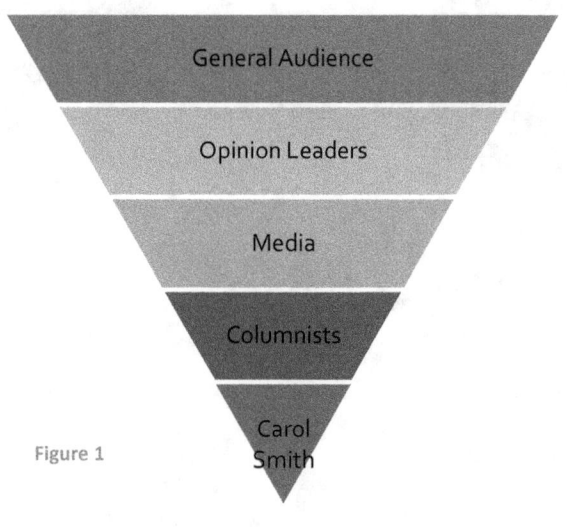

Figure 1

Though you will certainly be able to reach a target audience far greater than one person, going through this exercise allows you to research the characteristics, concerns and knowledge base of a broader audience for whom that individual is a good representative. It is far easier to research what one individual thinks about your issue than a group of 500.

Figure one shows the progression from a broad, unfocused target audience to one specific person, a hypothetical character named Carol Smith. For the purpose of illustrating this process, let's say that Carol Smith is a columnist for the New York Times who primarily writes about women's issues, volunteers at a woman's shelter, and she has 300,000 followers on Twitter.

National Center for Injury Prevention and Control

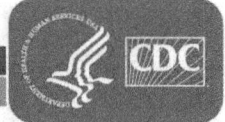

Step 2: Not a Popularity Contest

Effective communications is usually not about raw numbers. It is often about targeting key constituencies and influencing their behavior and attitudes to create change. It is often better to find and inspire a few committed activists than have 100 inconsistent supporters. For example, earning attention (and possible media coverage) from Carol Smith will have greater effect on your cause than getting 100 people to "like" your page on Facebook. In fact, the former may achieve the latter all on its own.

Step 3: Find the "Friend of a Friend"

Sometimes you may not be the best messenger for your message. Determine who influences your target audience and could help deliver your message with a better chance for success. Do you know anyone among that group? If not, branch out to "friends of friends" to widen the circle of influence until you find someone who can help you enter the "target circle" (see figure 2).

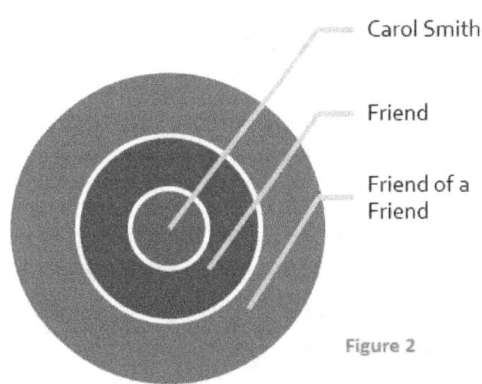

Carol Smith

Friend

Friend of a Friend

Figure 2

Step 4: Reach into the Circle

Once you identify an entry point into the target circle, craft a communications strategy that will allow you to move toward the bull's-eye. Be direct with people you know, and be strategic with people you don't know. If you know someone, contact them directly. If you don't know them use your target circle to determine who influences them, and then try to contact someone in an outer circle.

● Selecting Data Highlights

Since the NISVS report contains such a large amount of data, it will be important to identify data highlights that will be most interesting and relevant to the audience you are targeting. Though the data are not yet available, descriptions of the objectives and categories of data are available to help you determine which might be of most interest to your target audience.

The primary objectives of NISVS are to describe:

- The prevalence and characteristics of sexual violence, stalking, and intimate partner violence
- Who is most likely to experience these forms of violence
- The patterns and impact of the violence experienced by specific perpetrators
- The health consequences of these forms of violence

The NISVS report will present information related to several types of violence that have not previously been measured in a national population-based survey, including types of sexual violence other than

 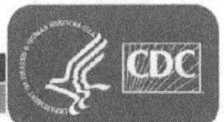

rape, expressive psychological aggression and coercive control, and control of reproductive or sexual health. The report will also provide the first ever simultaneous national and state-level prevalence estimates of violence for all states.

Specifically, the report will include findings on:
- Sexual violence by any perpetrator
- Stalking victimization by any perpetrator
- Violence by an intimate partner
- Impact of violence by an intimate partner
- Number and sex of perpetrators
- Violence over one's lifetime and in the 12 months prior to taking the survey
- Health consequences
- State level estimates

The NISVS data can be used for a number of purposes. First, these data can help inform policies and programs aimed at preventing sexual violence, stalking, and intimate partner violence. In addition, these data can be used to establish priorities for preventing these forms of violence at the national, state, and local levels. Finally, data collected in future years from the survey can be used to examine trends in sexual violence, stalking, and intimate partner violence and to evaluate and track the effectiveness of prevention efforts.

In addition to collecting lifetime and 12 month prevalence data on sexual violence, stalking, and intimate partner violence, the survey collects information on the age at the time of the first victimization, demographic characteristics of respondents , demographic characteristics of perpetrators (age, sex, race/ethnicity) and detailed information about the patterns and impact of the violence experienced by specific perpetrators.

Which findings you choose to focus on depends upon the interests of your target audience. Research your audience and see what specific elements of the report they would find most interesting. More technical statistics or data will be appropriate for medical professionals, scientists and researchers, while media outlets may seek a human story to bring the figures to life.

● Engaging and Communicating with Your Target Audience

In order to engage and communicate with your audience you have to first determine how they communicate and adapt your strategy accordingly. Are they Twitter pros, do they keep a blog or attend conferences? What particular phrases, statistics or data, resonate with them? What kind of language do they use? Understanding their behavior is crucial to effectively target and engage them.

Go to where they are.

National Center for Injury Prevention and Control

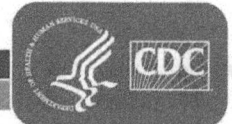

Don't expect your target audience to reach out to you for the information. Posting the information on your website or in a pamphlet at your location will only be effective if your target audience is already receiving their information from those sources. If your audience gets news from a few media outlets, try connecting with those sources to influence your audience. Search social media to get a sense of online conversations about your subject and discover links to other online sources.

Join the conversation.

If you want to truly engage your audience in a discussion, it is not enough to just present them with the report. You need to join their conversation, wherever that may be. Listening is an often overlooked part of a communications campaign. Listen to what your audience is saying and then respond with the information you want to share in a context that is relevant to their conversation. Figure 3 shows how to employ this strategy on Twitter. Simply blasting your information into the Twitterverse is not going to garner a lot of attention. Directing your comments toward a specific individual may yield better results. Sharing your thoughts as part of a conversation makes it more likely that your audience will respond.

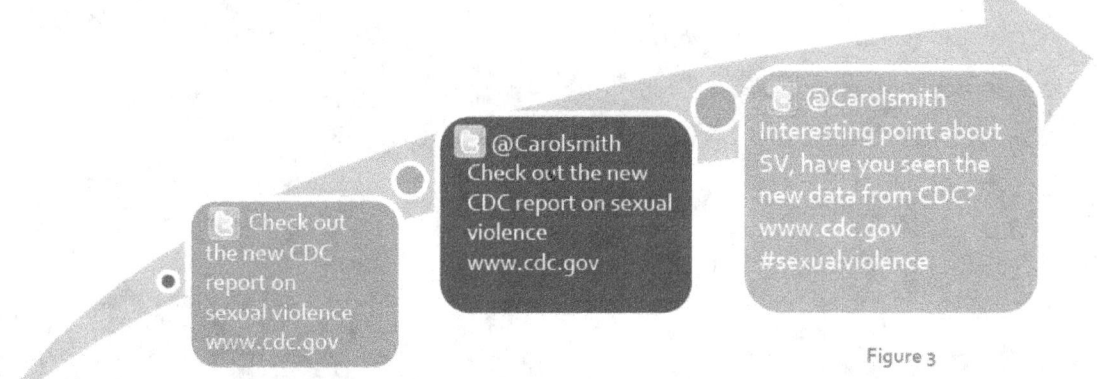

Figure 3

Use their language.

In order to successfully engage your audience, it is important to use the language they use. For example Carol Smith may only use the phrase "sexual violence," while other interested parties use "sexual abuse." Speak the language your audience speaks to increase the odds that your message will resonate.

Create Feedback Loops

Test the accuracy and effectiveness of your message delivery by asking friendly members of each "ring" what they are hearing? Do they understand your message? Will your target audience?

Adjust Strategy and Message

Communications plans are NOT set in stone. Media work is opportunistic. Change things around if your message is not getting to the target audience. Simplify your message if it is garbled. Communications plans should adapt to changing realities of target responses and opposition tactics.

National Center for Injury Prevention and Control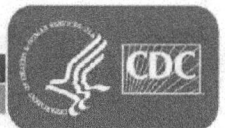

IV / Developing Messages for the *National Intimate Partner and Sexual Violence Survey*

IV. DEVELOPING MESSAGES FOR *NISVS*

Given the breadth and depth of data that *NISVS* will provide, it is important to start thinking now about how you will make sense of that information, especially as it relates to your cause. A message framework is an essential communications tool for distinguishing what information is most relevant to you and the populations you serve. Much like the metaphor it suggests, framing draws a border around the information you want to highlight and de-emphasizes the rest.

Consider the example below, in which the same image is framed in different ways, thereby conveying different stories about the same information. The picture on the left shows a pristine forest, conveying a sense of serenity. The picture on the right shows a wildfire swiftly consuming the landscape, injecting danger and destruction into the scene. Same picture, different frames. In this way, a message framework can create, or alter, the *meaning* of information.

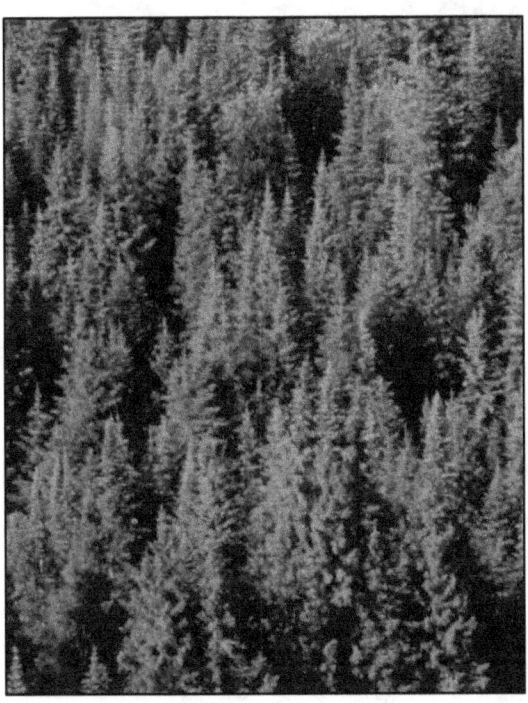 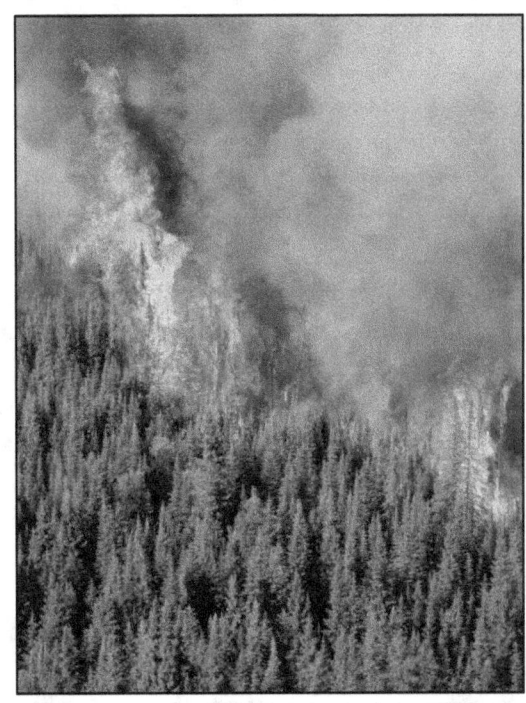

● How to Create a Message Framework

Before you create your message framework, determine these four things: 1) what you want to frame, 2) why you want to frame it, 3) who you want to see it, and 4) how they would talk about it.

1. What You Want to Frame | The Information

For a message framework to be effective, it has to be solidly grounded in the information it is framing. Though the NISVS data are not yet available, your experience in violence prevention can serve as a placeholder for this part of the process. Based on your experience, anticipate different scenarios – that the data will be consistent with your assessments and observations, or that the data will reflect rates that are higher or lower than you expect. Once the NISVS data are available, it will be important to ensure your framework has "proof points" in the data so that your messages are credible.

2. Why You Want to Frame It | The Goal
What is the outcome you hope an effective message framework would help achieve?

Now think of an onion.

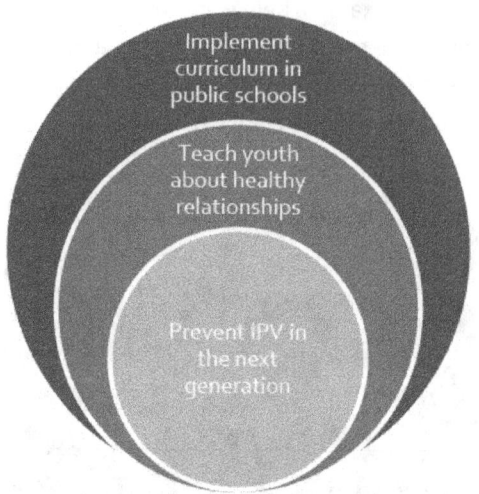

If the outcome you identified is a specific objective, like implementing a new curriculum in public schools, peel back a layer to determine the goal behind that goal. With this example, you might articulate that deeper goal as teaching young people the principles of a healthy relationship. Then peel back another layer to articulate the goal behind that goal – preventing intimate partner violence in the next generation.

If violence prevention was the first goal you identified, go through the same process in the opposite direction, getting progressively narrower in focus until you have identified a specific objective with a tangible call to action. Being able to connect immediate programmatic goals to a vision for broad societal change, and articulating the steps between, will lay the foundation for a message framework that can be specific or visionary. This will allow you to connect with various audiences according to where their values align with your goals along that spectrum.

3. Who You Want to See It | The Audience
To create a message that reaches and engages your audience, you need to know who your audience is. What makes them tick? What do they care about? What do they know about your issue already, and why it does or doesn't matter to them? It will be difficult to answer these questions if your target audience is too broad, because their interests will be too diverse, their knowledge of your issue all over the map. At the same time, you want to have critical mass to get your message to spread out like a ripple across a pond.

Much like the layered goals described above, your target audience may shrink or expand depending on the objective you're aiming to achieve. To get a new curriculum implemented in public schools, your target audience could be the school administrators responsible for selecting courses for the academic

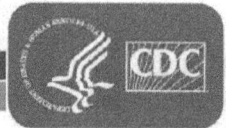

year. To teach young people the principles of healthy relationships, your target audience could be the high school student body in your municipality. To prevent IPV in the next generation, your target audience could encompass the entire community.

Different goals will likely have different audiences, and different audiences will likely need different messages to become interested and engaged in your cause. Refer to "Identifying Your Target Audience" in the previous section for additional guidelines on how to identify and reach your target audience.

4. How They Talk About It | The Language

One of the items you should research about your target audience is how they talk about your issue. Odds are good they talk about it differently than you do. The language your audience uses should inform the word choice of your message. Speaking their language will ensure that they not only understand your message but that it resonates.

● BUILDING YOUR FRAME

Now that you have identified the information, goal, audience and language that will inform your message framework, you are ready to build your frame. Like a picture frame, a message framework has four "sides": the value, the barrier, the solution, and the vision.

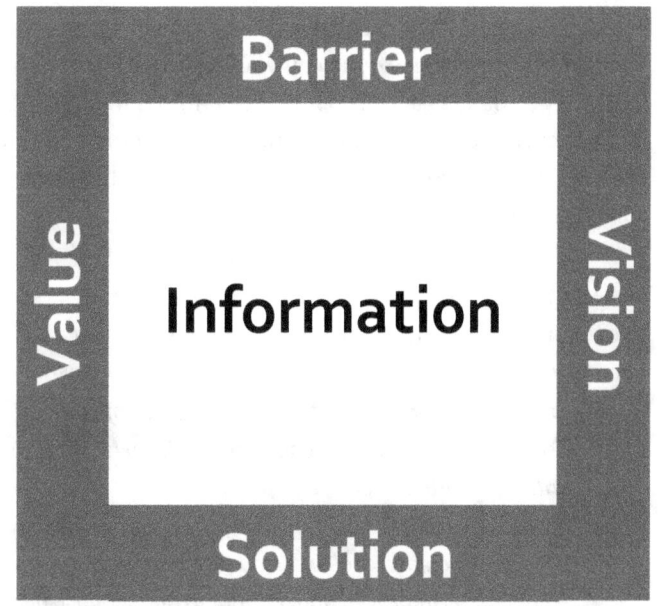

Value

Begin your message framework by articulating the value you share with your audience. It is a core belief that inspires what you do and why your audience cares. The value establishes common ground between you and your audience and serves as the entry point to the rest of your message. Returning to the example of trying to implement a new school curriculum, the value could be, "We want no harm to come to our children."

Barrier

Then identify the barrier that is getting in the way of that value. There may be multiple barriers to this value, so select the barrier that both hinders attainment of your goal and is recognized as a problem by your audience. In the case of the curriculum example, the barrier might be, "There is a common and dangerous misperception that children are too innocent to understand sexual violence. This does not match the reality of the situation and is magnifying the harm young victims are experiencing.

Solution

Next propose a solution that will overcome the barrier and aligns with the work that you are doing to address the problem. Describe the solution in a way that will resonate with your audience, based on the research you did about why they care about the issue and how they talk about it. In the curriculum example, you could share data on the prevalence of violence among youth, the increased risk to young victims of experiencing violence again later in life, and the long-term toll violence will have on their physical and mental development. Will your audience be better persuaded by presenting these data as statistics or as a human story? For some, it may not be tolerable to think of children as victims of violence; for others, it may be the only way to make the statistics sink in.

Vision

Conclude your framework by describing a vision in which your solution removes the barrier obstructing the value. The vision is grander in scope than the attainment of your goal; it aspires to a better world. At the same time, keep it grounded in your audience research and the language they use to talk about the issue. In the curriculum example, if your audience is educators or school administrators whom you are trying to persuade to adopt your curriculum, you might describe the vision as, "Let education on prevention, not the impact of violence, be the lesson that lasts a lifetime." Once you have articulated the four "sides" of your frame, you can create additional messages based on each piece as well as a cohesive message that incorporates all the elements.

The *NISVS* Frame

The following message framework was created to describe why NISVS was developed and provide a general way to discuss the survey in advance of its launch.

- **Value:** *Everyone deserves to live a life free of violence*
- **Barrier:** *There are significant gaps in the existing data around sexual violence, stalking, and intimate partner violence.*
- **Solution:** *The CDC developed NISVS to better identify and understand the magnitude and impact of sexual violence, stalking, and intimate partner violence. NISVS has innovative features that allow for an improved understanding of the public health burden of these problems.*
- **Vision:** *When people better understand the nature and extent of these problems, they will use that knowledge to strengthen and support efforts to prevent violence before it occurs.*

Core Message

The four elements of a frame can be combined into a core message, such as this one for NISVS:

 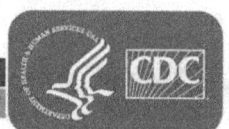

Sexual violence, stalking, and intimate partner violence are some of the country's most serious public health issues, but the good news is that they can be prevented. By better understanding the extent, characteristics and consequences of these forms of violence, we can take action to prevent them.

● *NISVS* Narrative

The core message can be expanded into the master narrative, which provides additional detail and context. Here is the NISVS narrative:

Everyone deserves to live a life free of violence.

Unfortunately, sexual violence, stalking, and intimate partner violence are some of the country's most serious public health problems. Victims of violence not only suffer the immediate injury but also long-term physical, psychological and social consequences. More than a decade has passed since the last major assessment of the prevalence of intimate partner violence and sexual violence, and there are significant gaps in the existing data on these forms of violence. More recent surveys have examined these issues in a crime or public safety context, potentially missing data from victims who may not identify or report their experiences as crime. The sensitivity of these issues has minimized some of the most serious public health problems in our country. Population-based surveys, like NISVS, are important because they help uncover violence that is often not reported to police or others.

When people better understand the nature and extent of these problems, they will use that knowledge to strengthen and support efforts to prevent violence before it occurs. The CDC designed the survey to maximize safety and to facilitate the reporting of sexual violence, stalking, and intimate partner violence using the best available knowledge and expert advice. NISVS provides the most current and comprehensive data about the prevalence of these forms of violence. It is also the first survey to provide simultaneous national and state level data. These data will help us identify who is most likely to experience these forms of violence and use this information to inform practices, policies, and programs that promote nonviolence and change the behaviors and environments that make violence more likely to occur.

With improved prevention efforts, respect and nonviolence will become the norm for individuals, peers, couples, families, communities, and society.

National Center for Injury Prevention and Control

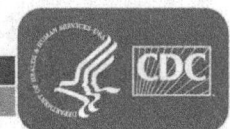

V / *NISVS* FAQs

V. *NISVS* FREQUENTLY ASKED QUESTIONS

In addition to the NISVS framework, core message, and master narrative above, we invite you to use the FAQs below to discuss NISVS between now and the November 15th release of initial findings. The following questions and answers are intended to 1) provide CDC's partners, grantees and other violence prevention organizations with additional information about the National Intimate Partner and Sexual Violence Survey (NISVS) and 2) anticipate questions that might be raised by various constituencies – such as the media, funders, collaborators, etc – and provide possible responses to those questions.

Like any resource contained in this toolkit, these FAQs are meant to serve as a general guide that you should tailor to your specific situation, needs and audience. The order in which they appear is not meant to convey their importance or predict the frequency with which they might be asked. The questions are organized by the following categories:

- General questions about NISVS
- Interpreting NISVS results
- Questions about specific NISVS findings
- Implications of the findings
- Background on methods of NISVS
- NISVS and other surveys
- Special samples (Military and American Indian and Alaskan Native)

● General Questions about NISVS

Q: What is NISVS?

CDC's National Intimate Partner and Sexual Violence Survey (NISVS) is an ongoing, nationally-representative telephone survey that collects detailed information on sexual violence, stalking, and intimate partner violence victimization from adult women and men in the United States. The primary objectives of the survey are to describe on an annual basis:

- The prevalence and characteristics of sexual violence, stalking, and intimate partner violence
- Who is most likely to experience these forms of violence
- The patterns and impact of the violence experienced by specific perpetrators
- The health consequences of these forms of violence

Q: Why was NISVS developed?

With the ultimate goal of stopping violence before it occurs, the CDC developed NISVS to better describe and monitor the magnitude of sexual violence, stalking, and intimate partner violence in the United States. Timely and reliable data on these forms of violence can be used to inform policies and programs, establish priorities at the national, state, and local level, and, overtime, can be used to track progress in preventing these forms of violence.

National Center for Injury Prevention and Control

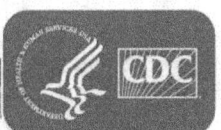

Q: Why is the CDC conducting this survey? Isn't disease control its focus?

CDC's mission extends well beyond control of contagious diseases. The CDC makes sure people and communities have the expertise, information and tools they need to protect their health. While just 30 years ago the words "violence" and "health" were rarely used in the same sentence, violence is now widely recognized as a public health problem, both because of the immediate injury risk as well as the serious long-term health consequences that often result. Violence also indirectly affects health in communities by reducing productivity, decreasing property values and disrupting social services.

Q: Why is this issue important?

The private nature of these public health problems makes them more challenging to monitor, evaluate and address than most other issues. But the need is especially acute because sexual violence, stalking, and intimate partner violence can create a ripple effect of health consequences well beyond the immediate injury. We've only begun to understand the cumulative health and social costs of these problems; conservative estimates begin in the billions of dollars in terms of lost productivity, direct medical care, ongoing health care and lost earnings by victims of intimate partner and sexual violence. Most importantly, these problems are *preventable*. NISVS aims to create a better understanding of the prevalence, impact, and health consequences of sexual violence, stalking, and intimate partner violence, so that we can inform and improve prevention efforts.

Q: What makes NISVS unique?

NISVS is the first ongoing survey dedicated solely to describing and monitoring these forms of violence as public health issues. It also includes information that has not previously been measured in a national population-based survey, such as types of sexual violence other than rape, expressive psychological aggression and coercive control, and control of reproductive or sexual health. NISVS is also the first survey to provide national and state-level data on sexual violence, stalking, and intimate partner violence.

Q: Who was surveyed?

The NISVS 2010 Summary Report presents data from the first year of data collection, based on 16,507 completed interviews (9,086 women and 7,421 men) in the general population sample. In 2010, NISVS was also conducted with a separate sample of self-identified American Indian and Alaska Native people, and a separate random sample of female active duty military and female spouses of active duty military. The results from these other samples will be provided in separate reports.

Q: How much state-level information is available in this first report?

The 2010 Summary Report includes data that was statistically reliable for individual states. For women, state-level estimates are provided for rape, sexual violence other than rape, intimate partner violence, and IPV-related impacts. For men, state-level prevalence estimates are provided for sexual violence other than rape and intimate partner violence. Information on the other forms of violence for men (e.g.,

 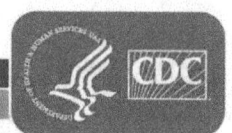

rape, stalking) are not included in this first report because the estimates were not statistically reliable. All of the estimates included in the state tables are for victimization over one's lifetime. State-level information for victimization in the year preceding the survey is also not included in the first report. Similar to certain types of victimization for men, we need to pool data across a few years in order to be able to provide reliable annual estimates.

Q: How should state data be used?
The state data are provided for individual states to better understand the number of people with victimization histories currently residing in a state and the burden of these kinds of violence on their population. Over time, NISVS will be able to combine multiple years of data to create reliable state-level estimates that provide information about more recent (as opposed to lifetime) victimization experiences among residents in a particular state. These data will be useful to inform prevention planning, program evaluation, resource allocation, and other efforts to address prevention and response associated with sexual violence, stalking and intimate partner violence.

● Interpreting NISVS Results

Q: Did NISVS make statistical comparisons between demographic groups (e.g., sex or race/ethnicity of the respondent)?
Formal statistical comparisons between demographic groups were not included in the summary report. Tests to determine which prevalence estimates differ significantly will be incorporated in future reports focused on the three main types of violence — sexual violence, stalking, and intimate partner violence. The reader is cautioned against making comparisons across groups because apparent variation in estimates might not reflect statistically meaningful differences.

Q: What does lifetime and 12-month prevalence mean? How should they be interpreted?
Lifetime prevalence is the proportion of people in a given population that have ever experienced a particular form of violence. Lifetime prevalence estimates are important because they provide information about the collective burden of violence within a population. *12-month prevalence* provides information about the proportion of people in a given population that have experienced a particular form of violence in the 12 months prior to the survey. 12-month prevalence estimates provide a snapshot depicting the recent burden of violence in a population. 12-month prevalence estimates collected over multiple years can be used to estimate trends in the burden of violence over time, suggesting whether violence may be increasing or decreasing.

Q: When comparing women and men, why do some 12-month estimates look more similar than lifetime estimates?
The pattern varies across forms of violence and the reader is cautioned against making comparisons across groups because apparent variation in estimates might not reflect statistically meaningful differences. It is important to consider patterns in the types of violence, the severity, the overlap and

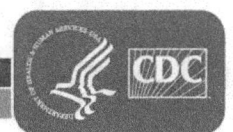

the impacts. Another point to consider is the relative difference in estimates. For example, the 12 month prevalence for any physical violence by an intimate is 4.0 for women and 4.7 for men and this reflects a 17.5% relative difference between the two estimates. However, the 12 month prevalence of severe physical violence among women is 2.7% and the prevalence for men is 2.0%. This represents a 35% relative difference in the opposite direction.

Q: Given the rates of physical violence reported by men, should we be doing more to support male victims?

It is important to assure that coordinated services are available and accessible for all of those who need them. The 2010 NISVS data shows that 1 in 7 men reported severe physical violence and that 1 in 10 reported an IPV-related impact (e.g., fear, concern for safety, injury, need for medical care or other services). The report also shows that, among the victims of rape, physical violence or stalking by an intimate partner who experienced at least one IPV-related impact, 75% were women and 25% were men.

Q: How meaningful are the apparent differences across states or by sex in the state tables?

It is important to keep in mind that the prevalence estimates are based on a sample and not a census of the U.S. population. Estimates that are based on a sample always include some error. This uncertainty or error is estimated with a 95% confidence interval. The 95% confidence intervals for the state tables are available online at (http://www.cdc.gov/violenceprevention/NISVS/state_tables.html). The confidence interval provides a range of values that likely include the true prevalence estimate. The 95% confidence interval means that we can be 95% confident that the true prevalence is within the interval.

Readers are *strongly cautioned* against comparing estimates across states or by sex. Estimates that have overlapping confidence intervals might not be meaningfully different from each other and additional statistical analyses are necessary to test for differences. Across all the tables, very few states have confidence intervals that do not overlap with those for the highest estimate in the table and even fewer have confidence intervals that do not overlap with the estimate for the entire U.S. population. Similarly, when data are available for men and women the confidence intervals tend to overlap and when they do not overlap the estimates are higher for women.

Q: Are the lifetime estimates by state meaningful if victims move from one state to another?

Lifetime prevalence is the proportion of people in a given population that have ever experienced a particular form of violence. The lifetime victimization experiences reported by individuals in a given state could include violence that occurred elsewhere. These estimates, however, provide important information about the proportion of women and men with victimization histories currently residing in a state. Given the potential long-term health consequences of victimization and the likelihood of ongoing health and service needs, these estimates can help states better understand the burden of violence in

National Center for Injury Prevention and Control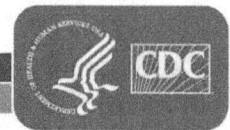

their populations. This information can also be used to inform prevention planning, resource allocation, and advocacy efforts.

Q: What does weighted data mean?
For NISVS, weighted data is the result of a statistical process that uses survey information gathered from the randomly sampled respondents in combination with national population statistics to provide data that are nationally representative. The weighting takes into account complex sample design features such as stratified sampling, unequal sample selection probabilities, and non-response adjustments. The technical note in the 2010 NISVS Summary Report provides more information about these features.

Q: How are weighted data interpreted?
Weighted data provide the best way to provide estimates that represent the nation as a whole.

Q: What are the strengths of the NISVS methodology?
One of the most important strengths of the NISVS methodology is related to gathering sensitive information in a safe, respectful, non-judgmental, and confidential manner from respondents and in a way that maximizes their comfort with disclosing difficult information. Other strengths include: 1) the ability to provide state-level and national data simultaneously, 2) the use of cell phone and landline samples because many homes now have only cell phones, 3) how NISVS moves beyond counts to provide information on the patterns, impacts, and health consequences of violence, and 4) the fact that NISVS is administered in a health context rather than a crime context because people are more willing to disclose victimization if they don't have to label it as a crime - particularly violence by intimate partners or family members.

Q: What are the limitations of the NISVS methodology?
NISVS relies on self-reports of victimization experiences. Despite efforts to make respondents feel comfortable and safe, it is possible that some victims were unwilling or unable to report their experiences. For example victims who are experiencing a high level of fear or coercive control in their current intimate relationship might be unable or unwilling to talk to an interviewer. Other victims, particularly those who were victimized a long time ago, might not remember some experiences.

Other limitations relate to the sample size. Although NISVS includes over 16,000 respondents, it is not yet large enough to provide estimates that are statistically reliable for all forms of violence experienced in the past 12 months or estimates for every variable for every state.

Readers are also cautioned against making comparisons across groups or across states because apparent variation in estimates might not reflect statistically meaningful differences.

National Center for Injury Prevention and Control

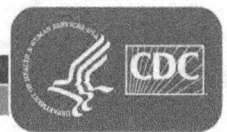

Q: Can NISVS results be compared to data from other surveys to assess changes over time?
This is the first year that NISVS has been conducted, so there are not yet multiple years of data available with which to compare rates. Because NISVS uses a different methodology than other current surveys that collect data on sexual violence, stalking, or intimate partner violence, results between surveys likely vary due to methodological differences and should not be interpreted as changes over time.

Q: Why are some groups more or less likely to experience IPV, SV and stalking victimization?
Although no group is free from violence, consistent patterns have emerged showing that women, young people, and racial and ethnic minorities are the most heavily affected subpopulations in the United States. There are a number of social factors such as attitudes about violence, poverty and disadvantage, sexism and other forms of discrimination and social exclusion that contribute to risk for perpetration and victimization as well as stressors resulting from limited access to education, community resources, and services that contribute to these differences. The NISVS data help us to better understand the variation across groups in the prevalence and consequences of violence but they do not explain why the differences exist.

Q: Can readers assume that violence *causes* negative health outcomes?
Beyond immediate physical injury, we cannot say with certainty that a past experience with violence was the specific cause of any particular adverse health outcome. However, these data allow us to evaluate whether victimization is associated with the likelihood that respondents will also report current health problems. We also know from other research that exposure to these kinds of violence can result in serious long-term physical and mental health problems as a result of the body's biological responses to trauma.

Q: Can readers assume IPV *causes* the IPV impacts that victims reported?
For the purposes of this survey, respondents were specifically asked questions about what happened to them *because* of what a specific perpetrator did to them. Therefore, the respondent, who is the best source of this information, has made a causal link. The impact measure includes all victimization experiences by an intimate partner that we asked about (sexual violence, physical violence, stalking, expressive aggression, coercive control, and control of reproductive or sexual health).

● **Questions about Specific NISVS Findings**
Q: What does this report say about the relationship between the perpetrators and victims?
Across all forms of violence (sexual violence, stalking, intimate partner violence), the vast majority of victims knew their perpetrator, often an intimate partner or acquaintance. Perpetrators were rarely strangers to the victims.

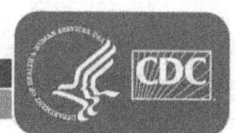

Q: **When are people most at risk for victimization?**
Although risk for violence exists across the lifespan, the majority of victims first experienced rape, stalking, or intimate partner violence prior to age 25.

Q: **Does this report show how both males and females experience violence?**
Yes, although women are frequently at greater risk of victimization and our findings are reported separately for females and males. For example, the results indicate that nearly 1 in 5 women (18%) and 1 in 71 men (1%) in the United States have been raped at some time in their lives and 1 in 2 women (45%) and 1 in 5 men (22%) have experienced sexual violence other than rape, including being made to penetrate someone else and unwanted sexual contact. One in 6 women (16%) and 1 in 19 men (5%) in the United States have experienced stalking victimization during their lifetime in which they felt very fearful or believed that they or someone close to them would be harmed or killed.

Q: **Do men and women experience similar levels of intimate partner violence (IPV)?**
It is important to fully consider the overall pattern of IPV experiences and this is one of the strengths of NISVS. While overall 1 in 3 women and 1 in 4 men in the US have experienced rape, physical violence, and/or stalking by an intimate partner in their lifetime, the contrasts between the experiences of men and women sharpen when we look at the specific forms of IPV, the severity of the physical violence experienced, and the impact of the violence.

Forms: While 92% of male victims experienced only physical violence, 36% of women experienced more than one form, including 12.5% of female victims who experienced all three (rape, physical violence, and stalking by an intimate partner). The type of physical violence assessed in NISVS ranged from being slapped, pushed, or shoved to more severe forms of physical violence such as being hit with a fist or something hard, beaten, slammed against something, choked, burned, etc..

Severity: While about 30% of women and 26% of men reported being slapped, pushed, or shoved by an intimate partner, 24% of women and 14% of men reported severe physical violence.

Impact: The types and severity of violence experienced contribute to the impact. About 3 in 10 women and 1 in 10 men experience these forms of violence AND reported at least one IPV-related impact. This means that, among victims, over 80% of women who reported rape, physical violence, and/ or stalking by an intimate partner also reported one or more negative impacts (e.g., fear, injury, missed school/ work, etc), whereas, about 35% of men who experienced these forms of violence by an intimate reported an impact.

Q: **Does the report include information about the sex of the perpetrators?**
This report does include information about the sex of the perpetrators. For example, the report documents that male rape victims and male victims of non-contact unwanted sexual experiences reported predominantly male perpetrators. Also, nearly half of all male stalking victims reported

National Center for Injury Prevention and Control

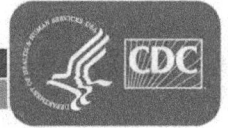

perpetration by a male. Male victims of other forms of violence reported predominantly female perpetrators. The majority of female victims reported victimization by a male perpetrator.

Implications of the Findings
Q: What are the implications of the NISVS data for prevention and services?
We hope these data will be used as a call to action for practitioners, researchers, and policy makers to engage in an array of activities ranging from prevention and intervention, to building the body of research. For example, the field can work to:

- Implement prevention approaches that promote healthy, respectful relationships and address beliefs/ attitudes/ messages that condone, encourage, or facilitate intimate partner violence, sexual violence, and stalking. These results underscore the need to focus on reducing violence earlier in life with both boys and girls, with the ultimate goal of preventing all of these types of violence before they start.

- Ensure appropriate response by ensuring access to services and resources and providing survivors with a system of care to ensure healing and prevent recurrence of victimization. An important aspect of public health practice is to tailor efforts to help those most at risk of victimization, and these data would suggest women in particular are heavily affected, as well as racial/ethnic minorities and younger populations. This suggests the need to address these disparities and provide needed services for victims, particularly those experiencing an array of consequences.

- Hold perpetrators accountable. Survivors may be reluctant to disclose their victimization for a variety of reasons including shame, embarrassment, fear of retribution from perpetrators, or a belief that they may not receive support from law enforcement. Laws may also not be enforced adequately or consistently. It is important to enhance training efforts within the criminal justice system to better engage and support survivors and thus hold perpetrators more accountable.

Q: What is CDC doing to address this problem?
CDC focuses on preventing sexual violence and intimate partner violence before it happens. CDC's work focuses on three areas: 1) understanding the problem—NISVS is a key component of this work, 2) identifying effective interventions, and 3) ensuring that states and communities have the capacity and resources to implement prevention approaches based on the best available evidence.

Some examples of CDC's work to:
Understand the problem
- Gathering information about sexual violence, stalking, and intimate partner violence victimization and perpetration through NISVS.
- Assessing the association between bullying experiences and co-occurring and subsequent sexual violence perpetration and to determine the shared and unique risk and protective factors for bullying experiences and perpetration of sexual violence.

- Examining the developmental pathways of violence perpetration, including those of IPV, among young women and men who have grown up in severely distressed neighborhoods in cities and who are now mothers and fathers.

Identify effective interventions

- Funding rigorous evaluations of strategies such as Green Dot and Second Step: Student Success Through Prevention to identify effective approaches aimed at preventing sexual violence before it occurs.
- Funding rigorous evaluations of other bystander approaches with campus and other populations and with different delivery approaches, including web-based applications.
- Examining an enhanced home visitation program to prevent intimate partner violence through a randomized trial that builds on the Nurse Family Partnership program.
- Conducting a randomized controlled trial to establish the impact of screening for IPV on health and quality of life.
- Developing and evaluating a comprehensive teen dating violence prevention initiative, *Dating Matters*™, based on the current evidence about what works in teen dating violence and sexual violence prevention.
- Rigorously testing the impact of family-based and dyad-based primary prevention strategies on the outcome of physical IPV perpetration and identified mediators with populations at risk for IPV.

Implement and Disseminate Effective Strategies

- Strengthening sexual violence prevention efforts through the Rape Prevention Education program by supporting strategies to prevent first-time victimization and perpetration; mobilize communities and build coalitions; increase awareness, education, and training; and operate hotlines. All 50 states have convened diverse sexual assault prevention planning committees and developed state sexual assault prevention plans to guide this work forward.
- Supporting the DELTA Program to develop primary prevention strategies to address intimate partner violence through funding, training and technical assistance. DVP funds 14 state domestic violence coalitions, which support local communities to implement and evaluate prevention programs while increasing sustainability.

CDC also collaborates with other parts of the federal government that provide leadership and resources for service provision.

Q: Are sexual violence, stalking, and intimate partner violence *really* public health problems?
Injuries and violence are widespread in society. Many people accept them as fate or as "part of life," but the fact is that most events resulting in injury, death or disability are predictable and therefore

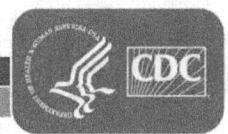

National Center for Injury Prevention and Control

preventable. The burden of injury and violence coupled with the enormous cost of these problems to society make them a pressing public health concern.

Q: How can we use these data to inform our work?
NISVS data can be used to support a wide array of violence prevention efforts, including:
- create awareness of these forms of violence within states
- inform local staff development and training programs
- set and monitor program goals at the state level
- inform prevention planning and priority-setting processes
- inform health education and other prevention programs
- support health-related policy
- inform funding decisions for state-level initiatives

● Background on the Methods of NISVS

Q: How are people selected?
Respondents are randomly selected through random-digit dialing of both landline and cell phone numbers. One respondent is randomly selected from the households. These people complete the interview over the phone with a specially trained interviewer.

Q: How long do the interviews take to complete?
The median length of the interview is about 25 minutes.

Q: How does CDC/NISVS measure sexual violence, stalking, and IPV victimization?
The survey asks approximately 60 "behaviorally specific" questions to assess sexual violence, stalking, and intimate partner violence over the lifetime and during the 12 months prior to the interview. By "behaviorally specific" we mean that rather than using general terms like "abuse" or "rape" that might have different meanings to people or be stigmatizing, respondents are asked about specific behaviors. For example physical violence includes behaviors such as slapping, kicking, and choking. Rape is assessed with specific questions such as the number of times someone used physical force or threats to make you have vaginal sex. A list of the victimization questions used in the survey can be found in Appendix C.

Q: What information does NISVS collect that relates to the context of violence?
NISVS is designed to monitor the magnitude and impact of violent victimization and has been designed to be consistent with the way victims recall experiences of violence – all behaviors are linked to a specific perpetrator and all questions are asked within the context of that perpetrator. In this way, NISVS is able to measure the following:
- Patterns of violence, including:
  - the forms of violence experienced by a specific perpetrator

 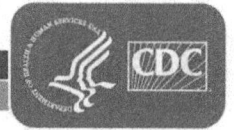

- whether multiple forms of violence were experienced (e.g., physical and psychological aggression, sexual violence and stalking)
- severity of violence
- duration of the victimization (e.g., the age when they first experienced any violence by the perpetrator and their age the last time the perpetrator committed violence against them)
- and frequency of the victimization

- The impact of violence by individual perpetrators (e.g., whether they were fearful, concerned for their safety, injured, had any post-traumatic stress disorder symptoms, had a need for medical care, missed days of work or school, contacted a crisis hotline, needed housing, community, victim advocacy, and legal services)

NISVS does not assess the context of discrete events (e.g., whether the violence happened in self-defense), but rather the overall violence experience as it pertains to a specific violent relationship.

Q: What constitutes severe physical violence and how does it differ from non-severe physical violence? What constitutes sexual violence and stalking?
The questionnaire includes behavior-specific questions that assess sexual violence, stalking, and intimate partner violence over the lifetime and during the 12 months prior to the interview.

Physical Violence. Physical violence includes a wide range of behaviors from slapping, pushing or shoving to more severe behaviors such as being beaten, burned, or choked. **The physical violence estimates do not include sexual violence.**

> *Severe Physical Violence.* In this report, severe physical violence includes being hurt by pulling hair, being hit with something hard, being kicked, being slammed against something, attempts to hurt by choking or suffocating, being beaten, being burned on purpose and having a partner use a knife or gun against the victim. While slapping, pushing and shoving are not necessarily minor physical violence, this report distinguishes between these forms of violence and the physical violence that is generally categorized as severe.

Sexual Violence. Questions on sexual violence were asked in relation to rape (completed forced penetration, attempted penetration, and alcohol or drug facilitated completed penetration), being made to penetrate another person, sexual coercion, unwanted sexual contact, and non-contact unwanted sexual experiences.

Stalking. Stalking questions were aimed at determining a pattern of unwanted harassing or threatening tactics used by a perpetrator and included tactics related to unwanted contacts, unwanted tracking and following, intrusion, and technology-assisted tactics. Stalking victimization involves a

 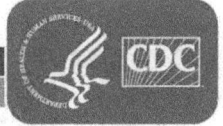

pattern of harassing or threatening tactics used by a perpetrator that is both unwanted and causes fear or safety concerns in the victim. For the purposes of this report, a person was considered a stalking victim if they experienced multiple stalking tactics or a single stalking tactic multiple times by the same perpetrator and felt very fearful, or believed that they or someone close to them would be harmed or killed as a result of the perpetrator's behavior.

Q: How is stalking assessed?

Stalking victimization involves a pattern of harassing or threatening tactics used by a perpetrator that is both unwanted and causes fear or safety concerns in the victim. For the purposes of this report, a person was considered a stalking victim if they experienced multiple stalking tactics or a single stalking tactic multiple times by the same perpetrator and felt *very fearful*, or believed that they or someone close to them would be harmed or killed as a result of the perpetrator's behavior.

The stalking behaviors assessed include the following questions about technology-assisted stalking:

- Unwanted phone calls, voice or text messages, hang-ups
- Unwanted emails, instant messages, messages through social media
- Spying with a listening device, camera, or global positioning system (GPS)

Q: What is meant by "made to penetrate"?

Made to Penetrate is a form of sexual violence that is distinguished from rape. Being made to penetrate represents times when the victim was made to, or there was an attempt to make them, sexually penetrate *someone else* without the victim's consent. In contrast, rape represents times when the victim, herself or himself, was sexually penetrated or there was an attempt to do so. In both rape and made to penetrate situations, this may have happened through the use of physical force (such as being pinned or held down, or by the use of violence) or threats to physically harm; it also includes times when the victim was drunk, high, drugged, or passed out and unable to consent.

Q: What is meant by "alcohol/drug facilitated penetration"?

This represents times when a victim was sexually penetrated but they were unable to consent to it because they were drunk, high, drugged, or passed out from alcohol or drugs. This includes times when a perpetrator intentionally drugged or spiked the drink of a victim but without the victim's knowledge, and cases where the victim may have voluntarily used alcohol or drugs, but the perpetrator took advantage of the victim when they were too intoxicated, high, or passed out to consent to sex.

Q: Will the questions change?

Potential changes to questions will be weighed against the impact on the ability to monitor trends over time.

 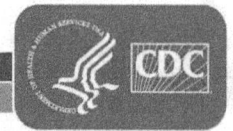

Q: How often are data going to be collected for NISVS?

It is anticipated that data will be collected annually through 2013 and beyond.

Q: How are respondents protected?

NISVS utilizes a number of strategies designed to enhance the safety of respondents and to improve disclosure and accuracy of reporting.

- Respondents are interviewed over the telephone instead of in-person to create a social distance so that they are comfortable disclosing their victimization experiences.
- Interviewers ask a series of health-related questions at the outset of the survey to establish rapport and establish a health context for the survey.
- Following recommended guidelines from the World Health Organization, a graduated informed consent procedure is used to maximize respondent safety, to build rapport, and to provide participants the opportunity to make an informed decision about whether participation in the survey would be in their best interest.
- The survey is administered by highly trained, female interviewers because previous research suggests that female interviewers put respondents at ease, which is very important for improving disclosure and reporting.
- Interviewers also establish a safety plan and follow established distress protocols, including frequent check-ins with the participant during the interview, to assess their emotional state and determine whether the interview should proceed.
- All data are kept confidential and private.

Q: Why doesn't NISVS measure the prevalence of perpetration?

NISVS is designed to monitor the magnitude of violent victimization and focus on factors most relevant to understanding the population burden. Victims are much more likely to disclose information than perpetrators. Data from our pilot study provided strong evidence that perpetrators are not reliable reporters of the violence they commit. Furthermore, there is a strong bias in underreporting, depending on the social acceptability of the behavior. For example, respondents are more willing to report that they committed psychological aggression (such as name calling) than they are to report perpetrating sexual violence.

Q: How can you develop effective primary prevention strategies if you don't measure both victimization and perpetration?

NISVS collects valuable information from the victim about the patterns and impacts of the violence experienced from specific perpetrators. Such information is necessary to make sure people and communities are aware of the issues, the subgroups impacted, and the health consequences. Bringing attention to this often overlooked public health issue is necessary to inform prevention policies and change social norms that perpetuate violence.

National Center for Injury Prevention and Control

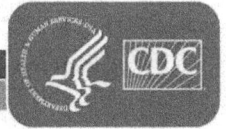

Q: What does the response rate mean?

The overall weighted response rate for the 2010 National Intimate Partner and Sexual Violence Survey ranged from 27.5% to 33.6%. This range reflects differences in how the proportion of the unknowns that are eligible is estimated. The weighted cooperation rate was 81.3%. A primary difference between response and cooperation rates is that telephone numbers where contact has not been made are still part of the denominator in calculating a response rate. The cooperation rate reflects the proportion who agreed to participate in the interview among those who were contacted and determined to be eligible. The cooperation rate obtained for the 2010 NISVS data collection suggests that, once contact was made and eligibility determined, the majority of respondents chose to participate in the interview.

While the overall response was relatively low, the cooperation rate was high. A number of efforts were made to reduce non-response and non-coverage bias. These include a non-response follow-up in which randomly selected non-responders were re-contacted and offered an increased incentive for participation. In addition, the inclusion of a cell-phone component provided increased coverage of a growing population that would have otherwise been excluded, including demographic groups with a higher prevalence of victimization (e.g., young, low income, and comprised of racial/ethnic minorities).

Q: Why weren't U.S. territories surveyed?

Providing consistent surveillance data for states and territories simultaneously with national data is a difficult balancing act which results in a complex sampling design. Due to limited resources, the first challenge was conducting enough interviews within individual states, to provide reliable estimates for as many states as possible, while also providing reliable national estimates. Similar to other CDC surveys, the intention is to add territories as resources allow.

Q: When will we have data for [state]?

In the current report, most states have some key estimates for sexual violence, stalking, and intimate partner violence victimization. Some states might require a few more years of data collection in order to ensure the estimates are reliable to report.

● NISVS & Other Surveys

Q: How does NISVS differ from other surveys?

Previous surveys have:

- Primarily been conducted within the context of crime or public safety. For example, the National Crime Victimization Survey collects data on the frequency, characteristics and consequences of criminal victimization. If a person is hit or punched by a spouse or boyfriend or girlfriend, they may not consider those actions to be crimes or report them as such when asked. NISVS uses a *health context* and victims of violence are more likely to disclose their victimization experiences when discussing their health.

National Center for Injury Prevention and Control

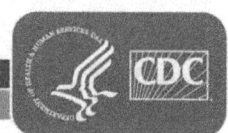

- Tend to cover only select populations – such school or college populations, or people living in particular states (e.g., state-based modules from BRFSS). NISVS provides both national and state-specific estimates. It's important to provide this information to states so that they can understand the magnitude of the problem in their state and use it for prevention planning and resource allocation.
- Tend to include a small number of questions. The number and range of victimization experiences included in NISVS is much broader than other surveys. NISVS assesses 60 different violent behaviors.
- Had different sampling strategies. For example, NVAWS, ICARIS-2, and BRFSS were all telephone surveys, but landline only. NISVS includes a cell phone sample because one in 4 adults in the U.S. now live in a cell phone only household.

NISVS is also unique because:
- NISVS is focused exclusively on violence; surveys that include modules or a few questions on violence and cover other topics in the same survey (e.g., BRFSS, ICARIS-2) typically yield lower prevalence estimates.
- NISVS provides both lifetime and 12-month prevalence estimates. NCVS, for example, only reports on experiences in the past 12 months.
- NISVS uses behaviorally-specific questions and avoids the use of questions such as "have you ever been abused"? Or "have you ever been raped", which are subject to interpretation by respondents.
- NISVS is designed to monitor the magnitude and impact of violent victimization and has been designed to be consistent with the way victims recall experiences of violence – all behaviors are linked to a specific perpetrator and all questions are asked within the context of that perpetrator. In this way, NISVS is able to measure the patterns and impacts of the violence.

Q: How do NISVS results compare to those from other surveys?
Given all the differences listed above as well as other methodological differences and differences in timing, it is not appropriate to compare NISVS results to those from other surveys.

Q: How is NISVS different from crime data on sexual violence, stalking, and intimate partner violence?
NISVS examines sexual violence, stalking, and intimate partner violence as public health issues, not as crime issues. To determine how these different contexts affect the reporting of sexual assault, the National Institute of Justice and the Bureau of Justice Statistics conducted the National College Women Sexual Victimization Study in 2000, comparing the methodologies of NCVS and NISVS. The study demonstrated that health-based, behaviorally specific questions, like those asked in NISVS; substantially increase reporting of violence. People may not identify their experiences with sexual

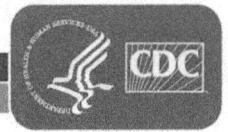

National Center for Injury Prevention and Control

violence, stalking, and intimate partner violence as crime, especially when it involves someone they know or love.

Q: Is this all the data that NISVS produced?
NISVS is a comprehensive data set with much more detail than could be included in this first report on the experiences of sexual violence, stalking, and intimate partner violence. Subsequent topic-specific reports of 2010 data are planned that will focus on sub-populations and examine each form of violence in more detail.

● Special Samples

Q: Didn't NISVS also survey the military population and American Indian and Alaska Native Populations?
Yes. In addition to providing guidance in the development of the National Intimate Partner and Sexual Violence Survey, the National Institute of Justice and the Department of Defense contributed financial support for the administration of the survey in 2010. The National Institute of Justice's financial support enabled the addition of a separate targeted sample of self-identified American Indian or Alaska Native people. The Department of Defense's financial support enabled the addition of a separate random sample of female active duty military and female spouses of active duty military. Data from these two additional samples are not presented in this initial report but will be described in future publications.

Q: Why was the Native American Indian and Alaska Native population a separate sample?
CDC and NIJ worked collaboratively to ensure a large enough sample size to produce reliable estimates among self-identified American Indian and Alaskan Native (AI&AN) peoples. The 2010 data collection included a separate sample of self-identified American Indian and Alaska Native peoples living in geographic areas with high concentrations of Native American populations. Similar to the general population sample, information from the AI&AN sample was gathered using random digit dial telephone interviews of the population aged 18 or older.

Q: Why was information on the sample of American Indian and Alaska Native populations not included in the report?
Only information from the general population sample was included in the 2010 report. This includes information from self-identified American Indian and Alaska Native people in the general population sample. To avoid confusion and to allow for a more detailed analysis of the separate sample, a special report will be developed through a collaborative effort between CDC and the National Institute of Justice.

 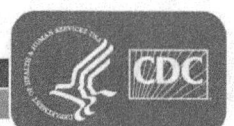

Q: Why was information on the military sample not included in the report?

The military data came from a separate, stand alone sample. Only information from the general population sample was included in the 2010 report. A separate analysis of data from the military sample will be undertaken in a collaborative effort between CDC and Department of Defense.

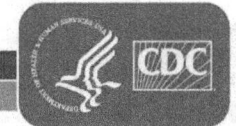

VI / Media Outreach: Generating Attention and Action around the Launch of *NISVS*

VI. MEDIA OUTREACH: GENERATING ATTENTION & ACTION AROUND *NISVS*

● NEW MEDIA: THE INTERNET AND *NISVS*

Over little more than a decade, the expansion of the Internet and the introduction of social networking sites, such as Facebook and Twitter, have created a major societal shift in how people share and receive information. According to the Pew Research Center's Internet and American Life Project, nearly 80% of all adults are online, up from 46% in 2000. Among teens, approximately 93% use the Internet, up from 73% in 2000.

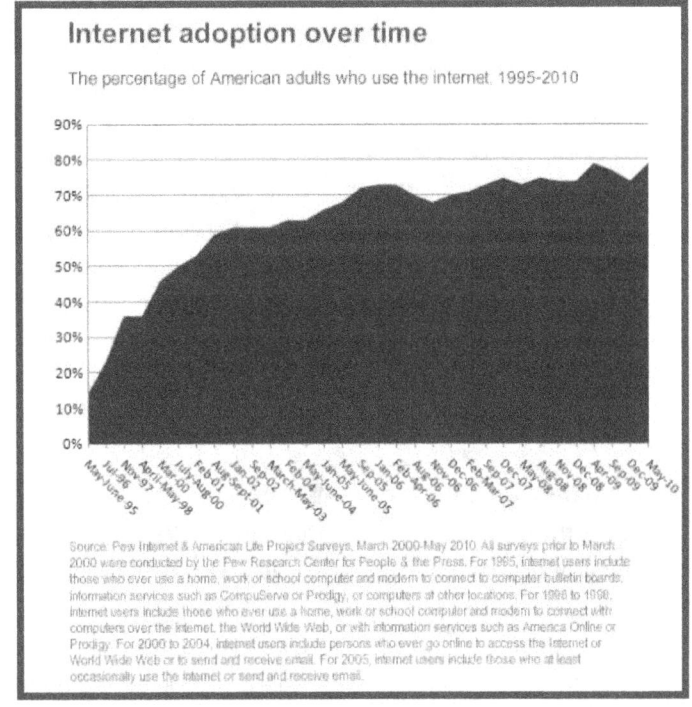

These new channels of dialogue have created a culture of openness that has affected not only our online lives, but our offline lives as well. The Internet allows people to create communities with others whom they might otherwise never know. It provides a setting where people are not limited by time or distance and where they can select their peers based on shared experiences, thoughts, and feelings. This may be important for victims of violence, whose experience may cause emotional or psychological isolation from the people physically around them. With the Internet, people can seek out online support groups, where they can create virtual identities in confidentiality.

The integration of the Internet in our daily lives presents a tremendous opportunity to create and participate in online communities that share data from *NISVS* as well as prevention strategies. The following sections provide information about online resources, present social media goals and strategies, and discuss how to make the most of your online presence.

● Online Resources and Tools

The following resource centers and websites provide valuable tools to use in online (and offline) communications campaigns:

- PreventConnect is a national online project that aids information sharing among persons and groups dedicated to the primary prevention of violence against women. PreventConnect offers

National Center for Injury Prevention and Control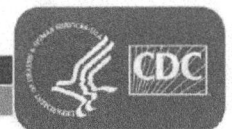

digital resources, including podcasts, interviews, a moderated e-mail list, Web conferences, presentations, and a wiki.

- The **National Sexual Violence Resource Center**, or NSVRC, is an information and resource center for all aspects of sexual violence intervention and prevention. NSVRC provides consultation, technical assistance, and resource development and dissemination. It has a vast online collection of publications and other information to assist those working to prevent sexual violence and improve resources, outreach, and response strategies.
- **VAWnet** is a collection of online materials to help individuals, public and private agencies, and communities put together activities to prevent domestic violence and sexual violence. VAWnet is a project of the National Resource Center on Domestic Violence , which offers a range of free, comprehensive, and individualized technical assistance, training, and specialized resources materials and projects designed to enhance current intervention and prevention strategies.
- **Veto Violence** offers online violence educational tools, including free accredited training; resources for program planning, creation, and evaluation; and success stories about existing programs and strategies.

● Social Media Goals and Strategies

"Social" is the operative word in social media. Like traditional media, social media are a means for communicating information. Unlike traditional media, which broadcast the news, social media *share* the news and engage people in discussion about it. Social media are more about conversing than reporting, about building relationships and recognizing personal experiences as authoritative sources of information and analysis. Social media allow people to communicate with one another in real time even when they are not occupying the same physical space. And when that physical space is dangerous, these sites can be especially important forums in which people interact and seek support.

Data from *NISVS* are certain to be conversation starters that present many opportunities to position your organization's social media platforms as the forum where those conversations happen. Here are some basic steps to create a successful social media space.

1) **Determine your goal.** The allure of social media often compels organizations to dive in before determining their reasons for using social media. As is the case for other areas of an organization's work, the first step for building social media presence is setting a goal. This goal should tie in with your organization's mission and broader goals while also looking forward to achieving a clear, realistic, specific objective and providing benchmarks against which to measure your progress.

2) **Identify your priority audience.** This is not "the general public," even if your ultimate goal is broad-reaching dissemination of information about violence prevention. Though it may appear counterintuitive, the best way to get exposure is to prioritize your audiences. If, for example, the mission of your organization is preventing interpersonal violence, identify the group most in need of

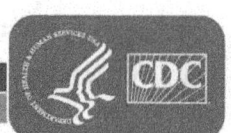

the resources you provide. Also identify who in those groups are the ones who lead change and get things done.

3) **"Listen" to inform your message**. To be able to reach your intended audience, you need to find out where their social networks are, what those networks are talking about, and how they're talking about it. This is where social media are different from traditional media. Social media offer you an advantage in understanding what your priority audience cares about. Conversations about your issue are the most informative. They illustrate what kind of messages will resonate and drive action. In addition to determining how your issue is being discussed, you can also identify where your effort may be misunderstood. This will enable you to prevent or correct misinformation. Think strategically about your audience and the best ways to reach them. Only then can you create effective messages.

4) **Create effective messages.** Clear goals and measurable steps toward them are supported by messages that resonate with your priority audiences. And that resonance is important. Messages are designed to achieve goals. A winning message takes into account what will work with the audience to build support. This does not mean restating your goals. It means making your case in a way that compels your priority audience to turn passive support into action.

5) **Evaluate your message.** In much the same way that you listened to your priority audience to inform your message, you can listen to determine the effect of your message. How are people talking about your message, your organization, and your issue? Has that conversation changed? Social media also present the opportunity to ask for feedback about your message and its effect on your priority audience.

● **Making the Most of Online Presence**
Social media are growing and evolving more rapidly than any other information outlet. Among the many channels are a few mainstays. Their staying power reflects their unique community-building qualities and outreach capacities, which you should take into consideration when identifying your priority audience and developing content.

Though your content should be tailored for each medium and audience, it should also complement the content on your other platforms. Here's an overview of best practices for creating a social media strategy that makes the most of your online presence. They will help make the work of your organization more transparent, accessible, and influential and allow you to connect with a wide range of people, regardless of time and location.

Your **website** is your hub. It's also the most static platform. It provides comprehensive information about who you are and what you do. Some of the content is probably dynamic, but your website's structure, purpose, and essential information don't often change.

National Center for Injury Prevention and Control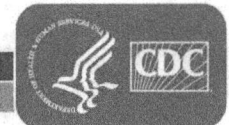

A **blog** is where we get to know the personality or editorial voice of your organization. The content is more dynamic and more personal than a website and can offer opinion and analysis. It's also a forum that allows you to respond to current items.

Facebook

Facebook is currently the largest online social networking site. It's designed for you to share content with your personal networks, although users can be selective about who sees their information. Whereas websites and blogs emphasize the organization, Facebook emphasizes the organization's network. This offers opportunities for social validation of both the organization and its fans through comments and the button that shows you "like" a post or a page.

At right is a screenshot from the Facebook page of the National Sexual Violence Resource Center, which shows successful use of sharing news that a) starts a conversation and b) invites the feedback of its network.

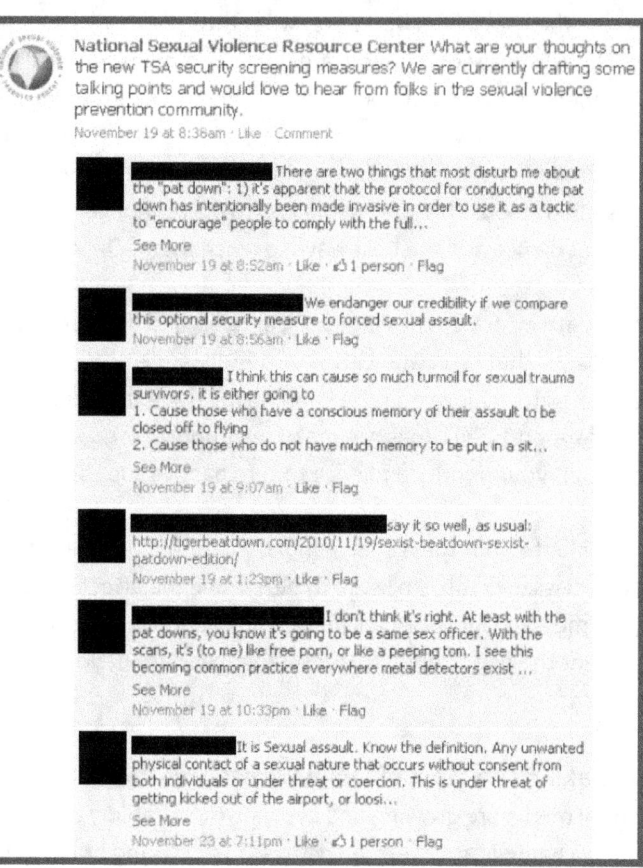

How to Get Started on Facebook:

1. *Go to https://www.facebook.com/pages/create.php, click on "Company, Organization, or Institution," fill out the short form, click "Get Started," and you have a "fan" page.*
2. *Find constituents and ask them to be a fan. When you post content to your Facebook "wall"—the main page on your organization's profile—it will show up on your fans' "friend feed," which appears when they log into Facebook.*
3. *Make sure someone is responsible for monitoring your organization's Facebook page, moderating conversations, responding to criticism, and posting content.*

Ways to Use Facebook:

- Share news articles and blog posts about your issue—people can comment on these as well
- Send action alerts asking people to call legislators, sign petitions, etc.
- Promote upcoming events

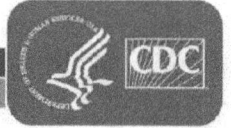

- Start conversations about your issue in the "Discussions" section

Some Thing to Keep in Mind:
- **Test drive first.** Use Facebook as an individual for a while to get a feel for what people share about themselves and their interests and how other organizations are communicating their messages.
- **Facebook is personal.** Allow your organization's fan page to have an editorial voice that sounds like a real person to take advantage of the personal appeal of online social networking.
- **Don't overdo it.** Send an update to fans only when you have an important question or important news. Otherwise just post to your Facebook wall. You will get a feel for the difference as you spend time using the service as an individual.

Twitter

Twitter is a rapidly expanding social networking site that is redefining how news is shared in real time. These instant shares are called "tweets." Like Facebook, Twitter is also about sharing content, but users cannot select who does and does not have access to it. Because users can easily follow and interact with one another, Twitter provides a great way for organizations to build and strengthen ties to reporters, bloggers, and thought leaders. Twitter users build influence by attracting followers through sharing valuable links; users also offer a fresh perspective on what they're sharing. They receive social validation on their tweets through "retweets" (reposting the original tweet) and replies. And they build a sense of community by interacting with followers on key topics.

Following is a screenshot of the Twitter feed for the California Coalition Against Sexual Assault, the handle, or username, of which is @CALCASA. The organization has well over 1,500 followers and has been "listed" 110 times, which means that 110 users have included tweets from @CALCASA in their own specialized news feeds. The organization's influence is also seen in the number of people who mention @CALCASA in their own tweets, shown in the screenshot displaying "Results for @calcasa."

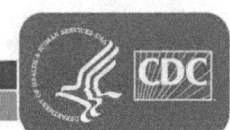

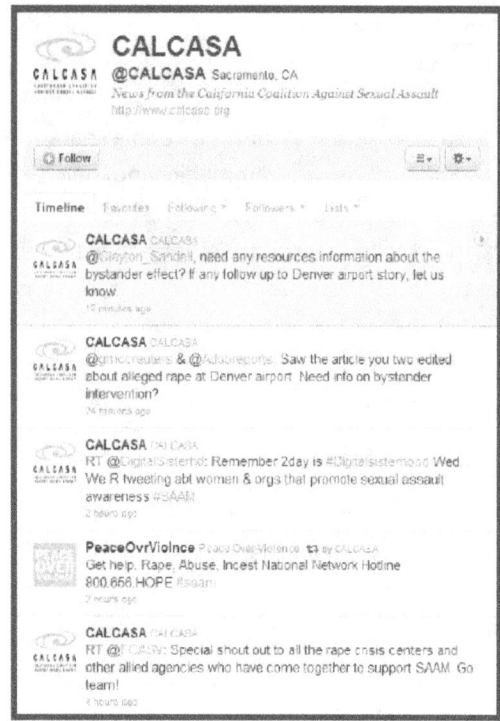

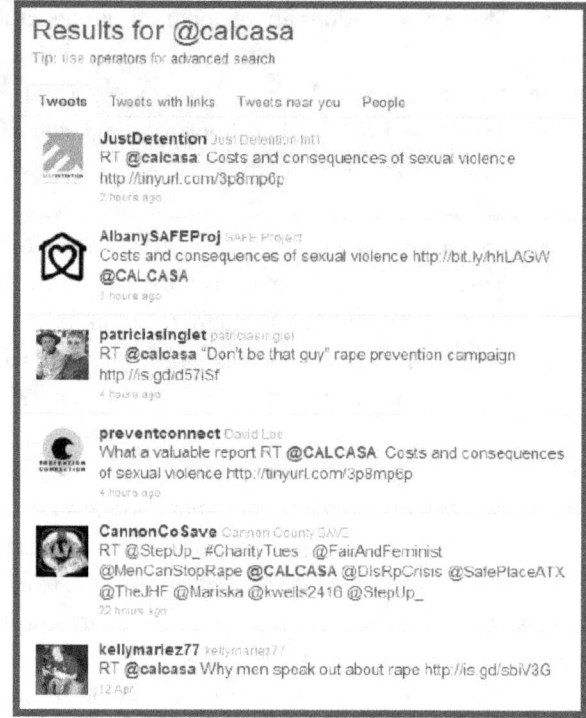

How to get started on Twitter:

1. Go to *twitter.com* and pick a Username—you don't want it to be too long, because the letters in your name will count toward the 140-character limit that others have for replying to your tweets.
2. Pick your password and answer the e-mail from Twitter. You have a Twitter account now.
3. Find people whose posts you want to follow at *twitter.com/invitations/find_on_twitter*.
4. Tweet by typing in the "What's happening?" box.

Tips for using Twitter:

- **Listen in real time** by following members of the media, officials, organizations, and individuals who are opinion leaders on the issues you care about. You can also search for key terms on Twitter at *search.twitter.com*.
- **Share links** to your blog or to news articles about your issue. Since Twitter limits what you can share to 140 characters, including spaces and punctuation, use web link shorteners like bit.ly (*http://bit.ly*) so that links fit into your 140-character tweet limit.
- **Interact by using @username** when referring to another person or organization on Twitter—then they'll see you're talking about them and can respond accordingly. You can also retweet, or share other people's tweets, by typing "RT @username" and pasting their tweet after.

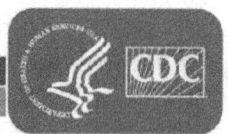

Examples: "I want to thank @Rainno1 for everything you do to help survivors!" or "RT @VAWnet An interesting report on the risk factors for sexual violence: bit.ly/abc"

- **Coordinate thoughts about an event or topic.** Encourage your staff to have Twitter accounts and use an agreed-upon "hashtag" (the format is #word) to tag tweets about an event, topic, or issue. For example, #VAW is a common hashtag to mark tweets about violence against women, as in "Thanks to our comrades in ending #VAW - @NNEDV @NCADV @CALCASA."

The CDC has developed a comprehensive guide to social media use, which you can access here: http://www.cdc.gov/healthcommunication/ToolsTemplates/SocialMediaToolkit_BM.pdf

● TRADITIONAL MEDIA

Building a solid relationship with a journalist or blogger can help to educate, inform, and inspire the general public about the overall goals of the *National Intimate Partner and Sexual Violence Survey*. While the media has the power to increase awareness and make political priorities of sexual violence, stalking victimization, and intimate partner violence, it is up to organizations like yours to educate and inspire reporters to cover violence prevention after the release of *NISVS* data in 2011.

● Garnering Media Attention
The following five steps will help guide interactions with media:

1. Research
- Read recent editorials in all local, regional, and national news sources related to SV, stalking victimization, and IPV.
- Read and follow relevant articles in academic or professional journals that touch on violence issues and prevention strategies.
- Look for articles and/or writers covering topics related to *NISVS* report findings that you want to further publicize.
- Contact the newspaper, journal, or online news outlet to find out who wrote those specific editorials; most outlets do not print the names of their editorial writers, but will provide the information if asked.
- Record the contact information of the editorial writer to pitch your news story.

2. Prepare a brief pitch to use when calling the editorial writer
- Put yourself in the shoes of the specific journalist you're targeting: What particular findings would attract their interest? What information is new or most relevant to the journalist's beat? How would they want the information packaged?
- Determine what the "news hook" is. What makes this information newsworthy and relevant right now? What other current events relate to this news or might be impacted by this news?

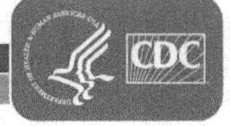

- Once you have this in mind, summarize your most salient points in a concise, attention-grabbing way.
- Get to the point right away.
- Don't spend time explaining the entire background on *NISVS*, just the points related to your pitch.

3. Plan and practice the pitch before calling

- A knowledgeable and conversational approach is best, so know your pitch inside and out.
- Know how your news relates to larger societal trends and public health topics, especially those previously covered by the reporter or outlet.
- Speak with confidence and emphasize the relevance and importance of your news to the specific person you're pitching.
- Help the reporter sell your story idea to their editor; can you connect it to something happening in your community? Another timely news report?
- Human interest: Many reporters look for the relatable angle to a story. Do you have an advocate, victim, or other spokesperson who can serve as the human side of the story? Being able to offer something like this may result in a longer article or more in-depth broadcast piece, versus a quick blurb with statistics only.

4. Call the writer or editor

- State the problem simply and briefly, and make a case for how an editorial or an article covering the findings could have an important effect on the audience.
- Stay upbeat, positive, and on-track with your message, no matter what happens.
- Inform the editor about prevention strategies, including why your news is important to discuss right now (for example, refer to the timely release of the data; the recent related coverage of IPV, SV, or stalking victimization; Domestic Violence Awareness Month; etc.).
- If your conversation is going well, ask for an in-person meeting with the journalist to inform him/her further about the broader issues *NISVS* covers or to offer more in-depth details on your specific issue(s).
- Be proactive: If you reach the writer's voicemail, leave a message but don't wait for a return call.
- Keep calling until a person answers; always ask to speak to the editor, managing editor, or issue-specific reporter/columnist.
- If one editorial writer or editor seems uninterested in your news, you can ask if there is another writer or editor who may be more interested.

5. If you haven't yet made phone contact, e-mail a short note that includes your pitch and/or relevant background information

- Use the same principles in your e-mail pitch that you use for phone pitches.

National Center for Injury Prevention and Control

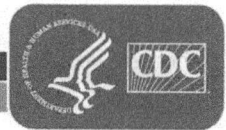

- Craft a simple, concise, and to-the-point message that will both provide useful information to the recipient and create a desire to know more.
- If appropriate, provide a preview of information you could share if the journalist is interested in covering content from the *NISVS*.
- Craft a simple yet compelling subject line that will stand out in a journalist's crowded inbox.
- Provide your contact information—e-mail, phone, mobile phone (if appropriate)—and emphasize your availability to speak in depth about your news.
- Be available: if you contact a news outlet, you should be ready to provide an interview at a moment's notice – and if you aren't willing to be the on-camera, quoted spokesperson, identify an alternate and make sure they are ready to assist.

6. Follow up

- Call the editorial writer, managing editor, and whoever else you pitched by e-mail a day or two later to see if they have had time to review your pitch and have any questions or need for further information.
- Offer any new information that might be of interest to them, especially that which is relevant to the day's news.
- Be professional, courteous, and persistent.
- Because they are busy, forgetful, and often overwhelmed with their ever-increasing responsibilities, it may take you several calls to even get on their radar.
- Don't give up!

● Engaging the Media

In the digital age, reporters, editors, and columnists are in constant need of fresh material to write for online editions as well as for print media outlets. As you know, *NISVS* data are fresh. So don't be timid about contacting journalists with story ideas or news of an event, recent societal trend, upcoming data release, or pending legislative action that may be relevant to your overall communications objectives.

Pick up the phone and also e-mail

Sometimes reporters may not be interested or will not have time to speak with you. Other times, however, they may very well find your story idea or news useful or relevant to their work—especially because this topic relates to a broad range of social, economic, political, and cultural issues. Regardless of the immediate response from the journalists you speak to, being proactive and contacting the media is a perfect way of putting *NISVS* and SV, stalking victimization, and IPV issues on their radar.

Build on the reputation of CDC and your organization

With *NISVS*, the CDC is providing important public health data on SV, stalking victimization, and IPV. CDC grantees can use the data as the basis for prevention strategies and programs. This provides a solid platform for your organization to credibly convey information that is serious, trusted, and

National Center for Injury Prevention and Control

newsworthy about SV, stalking victimization, and IPV. Use this opportunity to foster good working relationships with editorial, health, and policy journalists, positioning yourself as the go-to source for information about how the CDC data manifests in the field and informs prevention work.

Education

Good reporters and editorial writers are always looking for fresh data and news to follow. By providing them current, accurate, and up-to-the-minute information, it is more likely they will choose to write about *NISVS* findings and related public health issues than other topics. Educating reporters is important, because they might not know about your organization's role in preventing violence or the extent of SV, stalking victimization, and IPV in the United States. You can be a valuable resource for editorial writers by providing them with the information and background on issues in which they are interested. Whether or not they immediately cover your news, you can become a reliable source for future story ideas by providing useful information regularly.

Success

By following these steps, you are likely to generate stories about *NISVS* and your organization's specific communications and policy goals. Be assured, anything in the news mentioning IPV, SV, or stalking victimization issues, is an excellent opportunity to engage the media and promote *NISVS* findings. The following are some of the main tools for approaching the media:

- Editorial meetings
- Opinion pieces (for instance, Op-Eds)
- Letters to the editor
- Online commentary
- Media advisories
- News releases
- Calls to journalists
- Feature story ideas
- Press briefings (in person or online)
- Press conferences
- Photo opportunities

● Times When *NISVS* Data Should Be Especially Newsworthy in 2012

By planning media outreach around significant dates and events, it is possible to help focus the public's attention and increase the chances of gaining coverage for our news. Listed below is a calendar of dates that can serve as news "pegs" and should be used as opportunities to promote the campaign.

IMPORTANT: Letters to the editor and opinion pieces (for example, Op-Eds) are essential to promoting *NISVS*-related news locally and regionally. If submitting an Op-Ed, plan to have it completed at least

National Center for Injury Prevention and Control

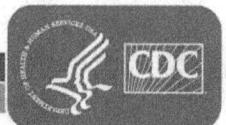

three weeks before the milestone day, week, or month to allow ample time to pitch, edit, and place the piece.

- National Stalking Awareness Month (January)
- V-Day (V-Day is a global activist movement to stop violence against women and girls. V-Day is a catalyst that promotes creative events to increase awareness, raise money and revitalize existing antiviolence organizations.) (February)
- Sexual Violence Against People with Developmental Disabilities Awareness Week (March)
- Sexual Assault Awareness Month (April) and Day of Action
- Childhood Exposure to Violence Prevention Week (April)
- Mother's Day (May)
- Father's Day (June)
- Domestic Violence Awareness Month (October)
- National Crime Prevention Month (October)
- Violence Prevention Month (October)

● 10 Tips for Preparing an Effective News Release

1. Make sure the headline, subheads, and first paragraph are powerful

The most important information should be in the first paragraph. Spend more time ensuring the headline and first paragraph are attention-getting and newsworthy than writing the rest of the news release. Journalists will look for the following in determining whether or not your "news" is newsworthy:

- Is it local? If it's a national or global story, what's the local angle?
- Is it something many people already care about?
- Is there important, new information?
- Is it timely? Does it have a sense of immediacy?
- Is there controversy?
- Is it unusual?
- Is it the first, the best, or the biggest of something?
- Is it tied to an important date or anniversary?
- Does it involve a prominent person or organization?
- Is there an interesting visual image that could be used with the story?

2. Put the most important information first

Use a "pyramid" style to organize information—featuring the most important and newsworthy information at the top and placing more general background information toward the end. If needed, provide links to additional background content, but don't count on recipients to read them.

3. Use quotations to bolster your news

National Center for Injury Prevention and Control

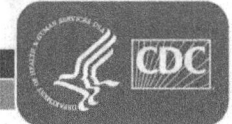

Aim to use a direct quote from someone, with attribution, within the first three paragraphs of the press release, and perhaps a couple additional quotes elsewhere. Using memorable quotes can bring the issue to life, validates the serious nature and importance of the news, and provides a platform to express strong opinions that the data itself cannot do. Remember, a quote is the only part of a news release that is reported word for word.

4. Keep it short
Keep the release to no more than one page, two pages if absolutely necessary. Rather than make the news release too long or complex, accompany it with a fact sheet or other briefing material.

5. Concise, concise, concise
Write short sentences of 25 to 30 words. Use paragraphs containing only two or three sentences. A good length for a news release is about 750-900 words.

6. Use a simple, concise news style
Avoid jargon, clinical or academic vernacular, and technical abbreviations.

7. Put the date and release details at the top of the page
State if it is EMBARGOED FOR RELEASE at a specific time and date, or if it is FOR IMMEDIATE RELEASE.

8. Conclude the news release
At the end of the news release, put END or ### to indicate end of the copy. Follow this with contact names, e-mail addresses, and telephone numbers for journalists to contact if they need more information from your organization.

9. Confirm that content and grammar are correct
Proofread the release carefully. Proofread it again. Send to a designated content approver for your organization, if necessary. Make sure all figures and statistics are accurate.

10. "Is it really news?"
Reread the release with one thing in mind, namely the first question a journalist will ask when reading it: "What's the news?"

 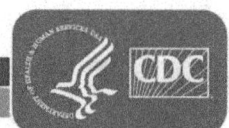

VII / Templates Section

VII. COMMUNICATIONS TEMPLATES

The following templates are meant to be tailored to your specific situation – the mission of your organization, the populations you serve, the data specific to your state, social and political environments, your relationships with opinion leaders, etc.

● STATE FINDINGS SHEET

CDC's National Intimate Partner and Sexual Violence Survey (NISVS) is an ongoing, nationally-representative telephone survey that collects detailed information on sexual violence, stalking, and intimate partner violence victimization of adult women and men in the United States. The survey collects data on past-year experiences of violence as well as lifetime experiences of violence. The 2010 survey is the first year of the survey and provides baseline data that will be used to track trends in sexual violence, stalking and intimate partner violence. CDC developed NISVS to better describe and monitor the magnitude of these forms of violence in the United States.

Highlights of 2010 national findings are available online.

[STATE] FINDINGS

NISVS also provides the first-ever simultaneous national and state-level lifetime prevalence estimates of violence for all states. The lifetime estimates presented for [State] provide an indication of the proportion of residents with a victimization history and the potential for ongoing health and service needs. These data should not be used to rank or compare [State] to other states, as the lifetime victimization experiences reported by individuals may include violence that occurred outside [State] and the estimates may not be meaningfully or statistically different from each other.[1] However, these estimates provide important information about the proportion of men and women with victimization histories currently residing in [State], which can help us understand better the burden of violence in our population and how to address it.[2]

- [Nearly/more than] [xx%] of [State] women have been raped in their lifetime and [xx%] have experienced other forms of sexual violence.
- [x] in [x] men ([xx%]) in [State] has experienced a form of sexual violence other than rape in his lifetime.
- [Nearly/more than] [xx%] of women have been stalked in their lifetimes.
- [x] in [x] women and [x] in [x] men reported experiencing rape, physical violence and/or stalking by an intimate partner in their lifetime.
- [xx%] of women in [State] who have experienced rape, physical violence, and/or stalking by an intimate partner reported at least one impact related to the IPV experienced, such as fear or concern for safety, PTSD symptoms, or injury or need for medical care.

---

[1] For more information about confidence intervals, visit http://www.cdc.gov/violenceprevention/nisvs/index.html.
[2] The report does not include state tables for rape or stalking victimization for men because the estimates at the state-level were unreliable (i.e., the relative standard error was greater than 30% or cell size ≤ 20).

National Center for Injury Prevention and Control

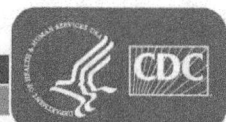

● **SOCIAL MEDIA POSTS**

Facebook: BREAKING: At 12pm Eastern Time, the CDC released findings from the National Intimate Partner and Sexual Violence Survey. The survey indicates that millions of U.S. adults are victims of sexual violence, stalking and intimate partner violence. Read the full report here: http://www.cdc.gov/ViolencePrevention/NISVS/ **Tweet:** BREAKING: @CDCInjury reports that millions are victims of sexual violence, stalking & intimate partner violence: http://www.cdc.gov/ViolencePrevention/NISVS/ #NISVS	Dec. 14th
Facebook: Yesterday we shared the CDC's new report, which indicates that 12 million US women and men were victims of intimate partner violence in 2010. This is a MAJOR public health problem, one we're committed to preventing. Click "Like" if you stand with us in this commitment. **Tweet:** New @CDCInjury data: 12M US adults per year are victims of violence by an intimate partner: http://www.cdc.gov/ViolencePrevention/NISVS/ #NISVS	Dec. 15th
Facebook: Knowledge is prevention. New CDC data shows that each year over 1 million American women are raped and more than 6 million women and men are victims of stalking. We are committed to reducing these numbers. Learn more at http://www.cdc.gov/ViolencePrevention/NISVS/, share widely, and click "Like" for helping stop violence before it occurs. **Tweet:** Each minute, 24 people become victims of rape, physical violence or stalking by an intimate partner in the US: http://www.cdc.gov/ViolencePrevention/NISVS/ #NISVS	Dec. 16th
Facebook: Last week, the CDC released data on the prevalence of sexual violence, stalking and intimate partner violence in the United States. The results were staggering. On average 24 people per minute are victims of rape, physical violence, or stalking by an intimate partner. Share these findings http://www.cdc.gov/ViolencePrevention/NISVS/ and click "Like" for efforts to drop this number to zero. **Tweet:** Nearly 1 in 5 women has been raped in her lifetime. Please RT: knowledge is prevention. http://www.cdc.gov/ViolencePrevention/NISVS/ #NISVS	Dec. 19th

● CHECKLIST FOR ORGANIZING A PRESS EVENT

Planned well, a press event can be an effective way to share new information, show broad support for an initiative, and garner broad media coverage. The new data from NISVS covers one base, the previous section of this toolkit covers another, and the guidelines below will help you organize an event that runs smoothly and effectively.

This checklist walks you through the steps of organizing a press event, starting four weeks out and working toward the event date. If you want to hold an event sooner, just condense the timeline and prioritize the elements that will ensure the most success for your event. Each item includes an italicized description, so that you can regularly refer back to this template as your event approaches and put each step into the larger context of event preparations

4 Weeks Out:

☐ **Determine a date and time**

Be selective. Choose a date when your event is likely to receive coverage because the issue is already receiving attention – National Domestic Violence Awareness Month for example. Also be aware of times when your event could be overshadowed by other events (ex: 9/11 remembrances).

☐ **Scout out a venue**

Choose a venue that is visually appealing and easily accessible for the press. Note: date and time might be subject to venue availability.

☐ **Secure speakers**

It is essential to have your speakers lined up as early as possible. Once you have a date and venue, you should proactively seek out speakers. The sooner you have confirmation from speakers, the sooner you can begin referencing them in press materials.

3 Weeks Out:

☐ **Build a media List**

Start by identifying the key outlets from which you would like to obtain coverage and build that list out to include outlets that seem likely to cover the event. Identify the specific journalists within those outlets whose work seems to indicate they would be interested in your event.

☐ **Solicit statements from speakers**

Gathering up comments from speakers prior to the event will help you to develop your press materials and, depending on what the reporter is covering, might be the difference between gaining and not gaining coverage.

☐ **Develop a media advisory**

National Center for Injury Prevention and Control

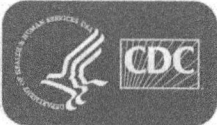

This is your opportunity to introduce your event to the public. You will want to specify event details and give an indication of why your event will be newsworthy to encourage attendance.

☐ **Develop visuals and/or infographics**

Visuals are one of the most important aspects of a press conference, especially if you are hoping to attract broadcast media. Think strategically about what type of visuals will re-enforce the message of the press conference and provide an aesthetic to be used in media coverage. Be sure to include your organization's logo on any visuals, including both posters and print-outs.

☐ **Check-in with speakers to see if they have any presentation needs**

See if your speakers will require flash drives, tripods or A/V set-up and plan accordingly. Maintaining communication with the speakers will also make them feel more invested in the event.

2 Weeks Out:

☐ **Send out the first round of media advisories**

Using the media list you built, begin emailing press advisories to your contacts. Make sure the date on the advisory is accurate and be sure to address the email to the correct person.

☐ **Keep track of any media advisory responses**

While not getting a response does not guarantee that press will not show, it is worth monitoring any feedback you receive. Doing so will provide a loose guide as to how many press kits to assemble, and it may also give you a sense of any questions your press advisory might leave unanswered. It is also a way to see what aspects of the event are most appealing to the press.

☐ **Write a press release**

This will be a more comprehensive version of your media advisory, written from the perspective of the event having already occurred. Adhere to the tone and format of a media story, but we aspirational too. Write the story you would most like to see a reporter write about your event. Take time to work on this and make revisions. Press releases are a huge resource for reporters and are sometimes re-printed in their entirety.

☐ **Make sure visuals and infographics are prepared**

Make sure that the visuals are in their final stages of completion.

☐ **Begin assembling press kits**

Print out press releases, statements from speakers, and graphics. Assemble them together in a folder. Be sure to provide contact information in case reporters have any questions after the event.

1 Week Out:

☐ **Send out the second round of media advisories**

Send the same advisory out as you did on the first round, but be sure to change the date. The purpose of this is to remind the press of the event, or bring it to their attention if they overlooked it in the first round. Follow up with phone calls to media you haven't heard from.

☐ **Contact the venue to confirm reservation**

The last thing you want is to ruin an amazing event by being without a venue. Call, email or stop by the venue to make sure that you are confirmed for the correct day and time.

Day Before Event:

☐ **Set up at venue**

The more you can have set up at the venue before the day of the event, the less you will have to think about. Depending on your needs and the venue, this can mean anything from dropping off materials to setting up chairs and podiums.

☐ **Make sure P.A. system is functioning**

While it is likely the venue will provide microphones and audio and/or visual equipment, it is still beneficial to make sure the equipment is functioning before event-day.

☐ **Send out third round of press advisories**

Drive the message home, make slight edits to emphasize that the event is tomorrow. Follow up again with phone calls to reporters who haven't responded to your advisory.

☐ **Print out your media list**

Having this on hand for the event will help you to identify the media.

☐ **Touch base with speakers**

If possible, have them stop by the venue the night before to practice speaking in that environment. At the very least, make sure they are still on-board and that they have everything they need to present.

Event Day:

☐ **Send out final press advisory**

Change the information slightly to reflect that the event is occurring today.

☐ **Arrive at venue at least 2 hours early**

Just to be on the safe side, give yourself time to make any last minute adjustments.

☐ **Hand out Press Kits to the media**

Press kits are essential to getting your key points across. Take note of attending press.

☐ **Be prepared to liaison between speakers and media**

Make sure to check the names of your media list as you hand out press kits.

National Center for Injury Prevention and Control

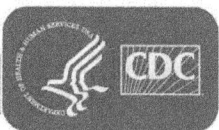

☐ **As soon as the event is over, send out press release**

Sending out your press release immediately after the event provides an opportunity for press who weren't able to attend the event to still cover your story. For press who did attend, it provides an electronic copy that they can use as they develop their story.

Day After Event:

☐ **Retrieve any remaining items from venue**

Pick up any materials that might have been left behind.

☐ **Send out thank you notes to speakers**

Thank them for contributing to the success of your event.

☐ **Be prepared to field follow-up questions from the media**

Be quick to follow up on questions or requests, doing so will contribute to the success of future events.

National Center for Injury Prevention and Control

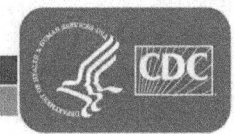

[Your organization's logo]

CONTACT: [Name]
[XXX-XXX-XXXX]
[Email address]

FOR IMMEDIATE RELEASE: [Date]

-MEDIA ADVISORY-

[Name of your organization] to share new state data on prevalence of sexual violence, intimate partner violence, and stalking

[Subtitle related to your organizations event, i.e.) *Coalition of XX organizations call on [who] to [do what]*]

[LOCATION] – [No more than one paragraph explaining what the event is, why you are having it, and the when and where details. and what you hope to accomplish]

WHAT:	[your event title]
WHO:	[your organization and partner organizations for the event]
WHEN:	[date and time]
WHERE:	[location]
VISUALS:	[description of visual elements to attract broadcast and print media]

###

[Your organization's boiler plate]

National Center for Injury Prevention and Control

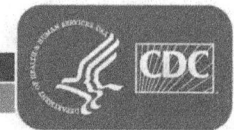